DIABETIC MEAL PREP FOR BEGINNERS

Healty & Delicious Meals to Cook, Prep, Grab, and Go - Diabetic Cookbook to Prevent and Reverse Diabetes with 30-Day Meal Plan + Special Desserts

CW00821723

TABLE OF CONTENTS

UNDERSTANDING DIABETES

Diabetes is an intense interminable condition endured by a large number of individuals around the world.

If you have diabetes and neglect to control your blood glucose levels, you are probably going to wind up with at least one genuine ailment, for example, coronary illness, kidney failure, and damaged nerves, among numerous others.

Pre-diabetes is a condition where your blood glucose levels are higher than they ought to be; nevertheless, not all that high that you are recognized as being diabetic. Research suggests that up to 70% of people with pre-diabetes proceed to develop full type 2 diabetes.

In any case, this implies that 30% figure out how to end the advancement of diabetes before it turns into a persistent illness. Thus, if you have been confirmed as pre-diabetic, developing all out diabetes isn't inescapable.

You can't change your past conduct, your age, or your qualities, yet you can change your lifestyle how you disport yourself and what you eat and drink.

HOW YOUR STOMACH RELATED SYSTEM FUNCTIONS

The foods you eat are, for the most part, a mix of starches, proteins, and fats in different extents. A bit of meat, for instance, contains, for the most part, protein and fats. Vegetables, for example, potatoes contain bunches of sugars.

When you digest a piece of food, it is separated into its key segments, carbs, proteins, and fats. These parts are then separated further in your stomach related system and are passed into your circulation system, which conveys them around your body.

Your energy originates from glucose. Glucose is only a primary sugar. Yet, it is your body's essential wellspring of vitality.

Most glucose originates from processing the sugar and starch in starches that you get from food, for example, rice, pasta, grains, pieces of bread, potatoes, products of the soil vegetables. The glucose created by processing in your stomach is then passed into your circulatory system, which conveys it to your body's cells.

Glucose is the fuel for your cells; it controls your developments, contemplations, and everything else you do.

To control your cells, glucose needs to get into them. It does this with the assistance of insulin.

Insulin is a hormone produced in the body It is delivered by your pancreas. The pancreas discharges insulin into your circulation system, where it goes around your body and gets together with glucose on a similar journey. The motivation behind insulin is to empower glucose to enter your cells.

To do this, insulin connects itself to a receptor in the outside of the cell. This causes the cell layer to permit glucose to enter the cell. The cell would then be able to use glucose as its fuel.

This glucose-insulin system needs to work appropriately if you are to be in control of blood sugar levels.

If the insulin doesn't carry out its function of 'opening the cell entryway' for glucose, the glucose won't have the option to get into the cell... what's more, the cell will come up short on fuel.

Diabetes is a condition where the glucose-insulin system doesn't work effectively.

There are two significant types of diabetes: *(a) type 1 and (b) type 2.* Over 90% of people with diabetes have type 2 diabetes.

In **type 1 diabetes,** the pancreas doesn't create any insulin or best case scenario, practically nothing. Type 1 can't be relieved. The primary way these people with diabetes can cope is by injections of insulin.

In **type 2 diabetes,** the pancreas produces insulin, which is discharged into the circulatory system. When the insulin shows up at a cell, it has trouble appending itself to a receptor. So, it can't incite the cell layer to open and permit glucose to enter the cell.

Insulin opposition is the condition where insulin can't connect itself to cell receptors.

Envision a key attempting to slide into a lock-in an entryway. The key can't get in if the lock is in a stuck state with a piece of chewing gum. There is nothing amiss with the key and nothing amiss with the lock. In any case, before the key can get in, the lock must be cleaned out.

One of the fundamental reasons for insulin opposition is having cell 'entryways' stuck with fat. The best way to 'unjam' them is to wipe out all fat beyond what many would consider possible from your diet for four weeks to about a month and a half (at any rate) until the cell receptors are liberated from fat.

So what do you need to do to prevent type 2 diabetes coming from pre-diabetes to the out and out incessant condition with its raised dangers of respiratory failures, strokes, visual deficiency, kidney transplants, leg removals, and other deplorable conditions?

CHANGE YOUR LIFESTYLE USING

HERE ARE 12 THINGS YOU CAN DO:

1) Avoid Stationary Conduct

A stationary lifestyle is one in which you sit a large portion of the day and embrace minimal physical activity. The connection between inactive conduct and the danger of diabetes is simply demonstrated.

An investigation of the consequences of 47 examinations found that individuals who went through the more significant part of the day occupied with inactive conduct (e.g., office laborers) have a 91% danger of creating diabetes.

If you work in an office, there are a few different ways you can change your inactive propensities:

- Stand up from your work area and stroll around for a couple of moments consistently.

- Stand as opposed to sitting when chatting on the telephone.

- Take the steps rather than the lift.

- Park far away from the grocery store, so you need to walk a decent separation to get inside.

- Go for long strolls at night (simple if you have a pooch).

- The ideal approach to turn around stationary propensities is to focus on specific activities you can do each day.

2) Get a lot of exercises

Studies demonstrate that physical exercise expands the insulin affectability of cells when you exercise; less insulin is required to empower your blood glucose to enter your cells.

Numerous physical movement types decrease blood glucose levels in pre-diabetic grown-ups who are stout or overweight, counting vigorous exercise, quality preparing, and high-power stretch preparation.

One study of pre-diabetics showed that high-force exercise expanded insulin affectability by 85%... while tolerably extreme exercise expanded it by over half.

However, this impact just occurred when they worked out.

Another study found that to improve insulin reaction in pre-diabetics, they expected to consume in any event 2,000 calories per week through exercise. That isn't too difficult to think about doing if you set your focus on it.

Try to locate a physical action you appreciate and can usually embrace, and afterward stick to it as long as possible.

3) Quit Smoking

Other than tumors of the lung, breast, prostate, colon, throat, and stomach related tract, just as emphysema and coronary illness, research shows that there are proven connections between smoking (and introduction to recycled smoke) and type 2 diabetes.

Smoking builds the danger of diabetes by 44% in regular smokers and 61% in overwhelming smokers (more than 20 cigarettes every day), contrasted with non-smokers as per a meta-investigation of a few studies that together secured more than one million smokers.

Stopping smoking diminishes this hazard after some time, but not right away.

An investigation of moderately aged male smokers shows that five years in the wake of stopping their danger of developing diabetes was decreased by 13%. After 20 years, it was equivalent to individuals who had never smoked.

4) Lose Weight

Most individuals who develop type 2 diabetes are overweight or hefty. Also, individuals with pre-diabetes will, in general, have visceral fat, i.e., they haul their excess weight around their center and stomach organs, for example, the liver.

Studies have demonstrated that increased visceral fat advances insulin opposition, expanding the danger of diabetes significantly. This hazard can be diminished by shedding pounds, particularly around the center.

One investigation of more than 1,000 individuals found that for each kilogram (2.2 lbs.) they lost; their danger of diabetes was decreased by 16%. This examination additionally found that the most extreme decrease of a hazard was 96%, i.e., lost 6 kilograms

(13.2 lbs.).

There are numerous sound ways of shedding pounds by exercise and dieting.

You have numerous dietary alternatives to browse Mediterranean, paleo, low-carb, vegan. The best, maybe, is the Beating-Diabetes diet.

5) Reduce the Fat in your Diet

As you know, the primary driver of type 2 diabetes is fat gumming up the receptors in your muscle cells, so the insulin can't open the cell films to permit glucose to enter. The "fix" is to unblock the receptors.

As you are pre-diabetic, fat is now starting to gum up the receptors. You can unblock the receptors by limiting the fat you ingest in your diet.

To limit the fat you eat:

- Make sure that under 10% of the content in any food you eat originates from fat (read the marks), and

- Reduce your utilization of meat, eggs, and dairy items, as reasonable, and center around foods dependent on plants (products of the soil).

- *It's that simple.*

6)   Reduce the Refined Carbs you eat

Refined starches are refined sugar and grain items that have been processed. The procedure removes dietary fiber, nutrients, and minerals from the grains.

Instances of refined carbs incorporate white sugar, granulated sugar, high fructose corn syrup, etc., just as white flour, white rice, white pasta, and so on. These are processed more quickly than complex starches.

Numerous investigations have indicated a connection between the constant utilization of sugar or other refined carbs and the danger of diabetes.

For instance, an examination that checked an aggregate of 37 investigations found that people with the most consumption of refined carbs are 40% more likely to develop diabetes than those with the least consumption.

This is because straightforward sugars and refined carbs are processed rapidly and are consumed quickly in the circulation system—this results in a spike in the degree of glucose in your blood.

However, as you are pre-diabetic, your body's cells are impervious to the activity of insulin. Therefore, the glucose spike invigorates your pancreas to deliver more insulin.

After some time, this prompts more elevated blood glucose and insulin levels in your blood until you develop out and out diabetes.

To keep away from this, you must stop placing sugar in your tea and espresso and quit drinking soft drinks and other sweet beverages.

You additionally need to begin eating regular foods, for example, entire grains, vegetables, organic products, and uncooked vegetables, which are all top hotspots for complex starches.

7) Eat a High Fiber Diet

Dietary fiber is the unpalatable bit of plant foodstuffs. There are two types of fiber and eating a lot of the two types is pivotal for forestalling pre-diabetes.

Solvent fiber will be a fiber that disintegrates in water to form a gooey gel-like material that eases back the rate at which food is ingested, lessening the probability of unexpected spikes in blood glucose.

Insoluble fiber can't disintegrate in water; however, it assimilates water, which makes your stool increasingly firm, facilitating its passing. It also is connected to decreases in blood glucose; however, how it functions isn't clear.

The primary sources of solvent fiber are vegetables (beans, peas, etc.) grains (oats, rye, and barley) vegetables, for example, broccoli, carrot and artichokes root vegetables, for example, yams and onions... also, the fleshy part of certain natural products, for example, prunes, plums, berries, bananas, apples, and pears.

Insoluble fiber is, for the most part, found in entire grains wheat and corn grain, nuts, seeds, potato skins, flax seeds. Also found in organic product, for example, avocados and bananas a few skins, for example, on tomatoes also, vegetables, for example, green beans, cauliflower, courgettes (zucchini) and celery.

A few plants contain significant measures of both dissolvable and insoluble fiber. Eating a lot of vegetables and foods grown from the ground will give you enough fiber to forestall your pre-diabetes developing into diabetes.

8) Minimize Your Consumption of Prepared foods

Prepared foods, for example, bacon, sausage, pâté, salami, breakfast oats, cheddar, tinned vegetables, bread, delicious tidbits (crisps, hotdog moves, pies, and pastries), cakes and rolls, microwave suppers, etc., are brimming with oils, including fats, included sugar, refined grains and a wide range of added substances.

Prepared foods are connected to a wide range of medical issues, including diabetes. One investigation found that low-quality diets that are high in processed foods increase the danger of diabetes by 30%.

So, to delay your diabetes developing into interminable diabetes, you have to decrease prepared foods. Eat vegetables, natural products, nuts, and other plant-based foods.

9) Restrict Partition Sizes

When food hits your stomach, everything begins to be processed on the double.

Along these lines, eating a lot at one sitting has been shown to cause higher glucose and insulin levels in pre-diabetic individuals.

A two-year investigation of pre-diabetic men found that the individuals who reduced the quantity of food they ate in one supper had a 46% lower danger of developing diabetes contrasted with the individuals who kept on eating huge amounts.

Another investigation of individuals with pre-diabetes inferred that the individuals who practiced portion control brought down their blood glucose and insulin levels significantly in the following 12 weeks.

Along these lines, to forestall the beginning of diabetes, you have to practice portion control.

10) Drink Lots of Water, Coffee and Tea

Drinking lots of water should be your essential drink.

Sticking with water more often means that you will keep away from drinks that are high in sugar, additives, and other harmful ingredients.

A massive observational investigation of 2,800 individuals found that the individuals who consumed multiple servings of sugar-improved drinks a day had a 99% increased danger of developing

LADA and a 20% higher risk of developing type 2 diabetes.

LADA, inactive immune system diabetes of grown-ups, is a type of type 1 diabetes that happens in individuals more than 18 years old.

A few studies have discovered that expanded water utilization (as opposed to increasing the number of soft drinks or natural product juices you devour) prompts better blood glucose control and insulin reaction.

One 24-week study, for instance, demonstrated that overweight grown-ups who changed diet soft drinks for water as a significant aspect of a health improvement plan encountered a reduction in insulin opposition and lower levels of blood glucose and insulin in the wake of fasting.

So, drink a lot of water, at any rate, 2 to 4 liters, a day to stop diabetes developing.

Ensure you stay away from the sugar-filled soft drinks and caffeinated drinks. Instead, when you need a boost, go for coffee or tea.

Coffee and tea contain polyphenols, cancer prevention agents that may secure against diabetes. Green tea additionally contains epigallocatechin gallate (EGCG), one of a kind of cancer prevention agents that has been shown to decrease the production of glucose from the liver and to build insulin affectability.

A few investigations have indicated that drinking coffee

consistently decreases the danger of type 2 diabetes by somewhere in the range of 8 to 54%. The best decrease in chance is found in the individuals who drink the most.

An examination of a few investigations, which included tea just as much as coffee, discovered comparative outcomes. This survey additionally demonstrated that the danger of developing diabetes was decreased the most in ladies (everything being equal) and overweight men.

So, it's a lot of water, tea, and coffee for pre-diabetics who wish to abstain from developing diabetes.

11) Take Day by Day Healthy Enhancements

Nutrition enhancement covers smaller scale supplements, for example, nutrients, dietary minerals, and unsaturated fats.

Vitamins are crucial for wellbeing. All nutrients can be categorized as one of two primary types, water-solvent or fat-dissolvable.

Water-dissolvable nutrients are on the whole of the B vitamins, besides vitamin C. These nutrients are not put away in your body, and you dispose of abundant amounts in your urine. Consequently, they can't develop toxic levels in your body.

Fat-solvent are vitamins A, D, E, and K. To ingest these vitamins, you need an amount of fat in your diet. Any excess amounts are put away in your body tissues so they could, hypothetically, develop to dangerous levels. In any case, this is incredibly uncommon.

Minerals are partitioned into two types, significant minerals and trace minerals.

Significant minerals are the minerals you need in measures of 100 milligrams (mg) or more every day. These minerals are calcium, phosphorus, magnesium, sulfur, potassium, sodium, and chloride.

Trace minerals are required in measures of fewer than 100mg every day. Trace minerals incorporate iron, iodine, zinc, fluoride, selenium, copper, chromium, manganese, and molybdenum.

Minerals are used in an assortment of functions. For instance, your body uses calcium to make bones and teeth, and iron to make the hemoglobin in your red platelets.

Although, everything being equal and dietary minerals are not yet entirely understood by researchers, and even though the results of clinical tests regularly contradict one another, day by day dietary enhancement should help forestall your pre-diabetes developing into diabetes.

This is what you must take every day:

- Multivitamin: to ensure all your dietary needs are secured.

- Vitamin B12 (4mcg) in a different tablet: for the wellbeing of your sensory system as your pre-diabetes is probably going to be influencing your nerves as of now.

- Calcium (400mg) in addition to vitamin D (2.5mcg) together in a different tablet to guarantee the soundness of your bones.

- High-quality cod-liver oil capsule with vitamins D and E, in a different capsule: to ensure you ingest sufficient measures of the essential unsaturated fats omega three and omega 6.

There is an accentuation on vitamin D because this vitamin is significant for adequate power over your blood glucose.

An assortment of studies shows that people who have too little vitamin D in their circulation system are at more danger of all types of diabetes. One examination found that people with the most significant levels of vitamin D in their blood were 43% less likely to develop diabetes contrasted with people with the least levels.

Most wellbeing associations suggest keeping up a vitamin D blood level of at any rate 75nmol/l (30ng/ml).

Controlled investigations have demonstrated that when individuals who lack vitamin D take supplements, their blood glucose levels are standardized, and their danger of developing diabetes is diminished significantly.

12) Add Characteristic Herbs to Your Diet

The web is loaded with claims, for the most part, fake, that specific herbs can prevent your pre-diabetes from developing into the all-out form of the disease. Here are a couple of the more believable cases:

- **Cinnamon**: is a profoundly sweet-smelling zest with an exceptionally particular flavor. It is used in conventional medicine to treat an assortment of ailments, obviously with some success.

Reports on the web recommend that cinnamon can cut fasting glucose levels by up to 30%, so I started sprinkling one enormous teaspoon on my porridge (oats) in the first part of the day. Inside a couple of days, my normal glucose levels on getting up had dropped by almost 0.5mmol/l (9mg/l) or about 8%, a considerable amount shy of 30% a significant decrease in any case.

So, I can't help suspecting that this zest, as ground powder you can purchase from your nearby general store, can help you improve your blood glucose levels and, accordingly, help prevent your pre-diabetes developing into diabetes. Bitter melon... otherwise known as harsh gourd or karela (in India), is a one of a kind vegetable-natural product that can be used as a food or medicine. It is frequently suggested for the control of diabetes.

Various clinical examinations have indicated that bitter melon is successful in improving blood glucose levels, expanding the discharge of insulin, and diminishing insulin obstruction.

In January 2011, for instance, the results of a four-week clinical trial were published in the Journal of Ethnopharmacology, which indicated that a 2,000 mg everyday portion of bitter melon significantly decreased blood glucose levels among patients with type 2 diabetes. Anyway, the hypoglycemic impact was not as much as that of a 1,000 mg for an every day portion of metformin, a well-known diabetes drug.

Even though it might be of some assistance in preventing your pre-diabetes deteriorating, the bitter melon should be treated with care as it has been related to unnatural birth cycles and actuated premature births in animals. Therefore, it ought to be kept away from if you are pregnant or need to get pregnant.

- **Curcumin**: is a part of turmeric, one of the fundamental ingredients in curries. It has anti-inflammatory properties and has been used in Ayurvedic medicine for quite a long time.

Research shows that curcumin can help decrease significant markers in people with pre-diabetes.

In a controlled 9-month investigation of 240 pre-diabetic grown-ups, none of the individuals who took 750mg of curcumin every day developed diabetes, yet over 16% of the benchmark group did. The investigation additionally noticed that insulin affectability among the individuals who took curcumin expanded, as did the working of their insulin-creating cells in the pancreas.

In this way, the advantages of curcumin in diminishing insulin opposition and lessening the hazard that pre-diabetics will develop out and out diabetes have all the earmarks of being very much demonstrated.

- **Berberine**: is an alkaloid extricated from different plants used in customary Chinese medicine. It is demonstrated to be mitigating and effective against diabetic impacts. It works by lessening the creation of glucose in the liver and expanding insulin affectability.

An amalgamation of 14 investigations of human and animal research has demonstrated that 1,500mg of berberine, taken in three dosages of 500mg each, is similarly effective as taking 1,500mg of metformin or 4mg glibenclamide, two well-known pharmaceuticals for treating type 2 diabetes. Berberine is one of only a handful of many supplements demonstrated to be as powerful as ordinary diabetes drugs.

Berberine, in any case, can react with different drugs and caution should be exercised... ask your primary care physician before you attempt to use it to forestall your pre-diabetes deteriorating.

- *Admonition (1):* Spurious cases that specific supplements can fix or forestall sicknesses flourish on the web. Anyway, there are a couple of reliable sources that contain research-tried data. These are for the most part associated with respectable colleges, clinical schools and teaching medical clinics.

- **Admonition (2):** Some herbs and supplements may combine with your diabetes prescription (counting insulin) and cause too low blood glucose. So, check with your primary care physician before using them.

BREAKFAST RECIPES

MINI VEGGIE QUICHE

A Veggie Diabetic Friendly Recipe. These are mini quiches that can also be called 'Stand Alone Meal'. It's easy to always have a delicious breakfast - ready to go. They are a great weekend recipe you can prepare for the family. You would love this meal because they freeze so well, and they can be served with a light salad and any of your favorite drink.

Enjoy!

INGREDIENTS

- 9 eggs
- 8 ounces of chopped spinach
- 1 small red pepper, chopped
- 1 cup of milk
- 1 cup of shredded cheddar
- 1/2 teaspoon of salt
- 1 small red onion, chopped
- Butter

PREPARATIONS

- In a large sauté pan, add a tablespoon of butter and melt it over a medium low heat.
- Add in the onions and cook until just translucent, for about 2 minutes.
- Add in the spinach and cook until it's wilted.
- Add the red peppers and more butter if needed.

21

- Sauté for about 1 minute and set it aside.

- Grease a muffin pan that holds 12 muffins.

- Divide the sautéed veggies between the tins.

- In a large mixing bowl, crack the 9 eggs and add in the milk and salt. Whisk together.

- Divide half of the cheddar cheese between the muffin tins.

- Then divide the egg mixture.

- Bake for about 10 minutes at 375 degrees F.

- Remove from heat and divide the rest of the cheddar, topping the quiches.

- Place it back into the oven and bake until the eggs are set. You can use toothpick to check.

- Remove from heat and let it cool.

- Serve and enjoy.

NOTE:

The mini quiches keep well in an air-tight container in the fridge for 3 to 4 days. You can easily reheat them in the oven (at 350 °F/180 °C for about 10 to 15 minutes) or in the microwave (on the high setting for 1 to 2 minutes).

PREP TIME: 15 mins

COOK TIME: 15 mins

TOTAL TIME: 30 mins

YIELD: 12 mini quiches

SHAKSHUKA

This kind of recipe is loaded with spices, eggs and tomato sauce. It's so easy to prepare and can be ready-to-eat within 30 to 40 minutes.

Using canned tomatoes for this shakshuka will be so easy (though you can always use your fresh tomatoes - it's not a problem). You don't have to worry too much because it's a healthy and diabetic friendly recipe you can always have in a bright morning.

INGREDIENTS

- 4 garlic cloves, finely chopped
- 2 teaspoons of paprika
- 1 teaspoon of cumin
- 1 medium onion, diced
- 1 red bell pepper, deseeded and diced
- 1/4 teaspoon of chili powder
- 1 28-ounces can of whole peeled tomatoes
- 1 small bunch of fresh cilantro, chopped
- 1 small bunch of fresh parsley, chopped
- 6 large eggs
- salt and pepper, to taste

PREPARATIONS

- In a large sauté pan, heat olive oil on medium heat.

- Add the chopped onion and bell pepper. Then cook until the onion becomes translucent, for about 5 minutes.

- Add spices and garlic, then cook for another minute.

- Pour the juice and can of tomatoes into the pan, then use a large spoon to break down the tomatoes.

- Season with pepper and salt and bring the sauce to a simmer.

- Make small wells in the sauce using a large spoon and crack the eggs into each well.

- Cover the pan and cook until the eggs are done to your liking, for about 5 to 8 minutes.

- Garnish with parsley and chopped cilantro.

- Serve and enjoy.

NOTE:

Shakshuka can be stored in the fridge for up to 1 week or can be frozen. To serve, warm in a pan with a little oil and top with the cheese / nuts / herbs.

PREP TIME: 10 mins

COOK TIME: 20 mins

TOTAL TIME: 30 mins

YIELD: 6 servings

HEALTHY GRANOLA

Healthy Granola is truly the best granola recipe! It's so easy and quick to make. It's delicious and flavorful and it's naturally sweetened with maple syrup. You can add in some possible variations to spice it up like dried fruit, chocolate chips and peanut butter or any other spices that you love.

Have this meal for your breakfast and be happy for the rest of the day!

INGREDIENTS

- 2 teaspoons of ground cinnamon
- 3/4 teaspoon of fine sea salt
- 1/2 cup of melted coconut oil
- 4 cups of old-fashioned oats
- 2/3 cup of unsweetened coconut flakes (or 1/2 cup of shredded coconut)
- 1 cup of slivered almonds (or your preferred kind of seeds/nuts)
- 1/4 cup of chia seeds (optional)
- 1/3 cup of maple syrup
- 2 teaspoons of vanilla extract
- 1/2 cup of chopped dried fruit or semisweet chocolate chips (optional)

PREPARATIONS

- Heat oven to 350 degrees F.

- Use parchment paper to line a large baking sheet and set it aside.

- Stir together almonds, oats, cinnamon and sea salt in a large mixing bowl until evenly combined.

- Stir together the maple syrup, melted coconut oil and vanilla extract in a separate measuring cup until well combined.

- Pour the coconut oil mixture into the oats mixture.

- Stir until evenly combined.

- Spread the granola out on the prepared baking sheet.

- Bake, stirring once halfway through, for about 20 minutes.

- Remove from the oven and add the coconut and stir the mixture well.

- Bake until the granola is lightly golden and toasted, for about 5 more minutes.

- Remove from the oven, then transfer to a wire baking rack.

- Let it cool till the granola reaches room temp.

- Then stir in the chocolate chips, dried fruit or any other optional add-ins you might prefer.

- Serve immediately or store in an airtight container at room temp.

- Enjoy.

NOTE:

You can absolutely preserve granola bars. You wrap the bars individually first with waxed paper or parchment paper, then store in large, labeled Ziploc bags. They freeze well for up to 2 months. To thaw, just pull out how many granola bars you want out of the freezer and leave them on the counter for 30 minutes.

PREP TIME: 10 mins

COOK TIME: 25 mins

TOTAL TIME: 35 mins

YIELD: 6 cups

CINNAMON OATMEAL MUFFINS WITH APPLE

Cinnamon Oatmeal Muffins are make-ahead comforting healthy recipe for people with Diabetics. They are awesome and can be packaged as snacks as well.

You can swap the apples for strawberries or blueberries and they have a subtle sweetness that makes a nutritious and delicious breakfast option for kids and adults as well. You need to try these muffins.

INGREDIENTS

Topping:
- 1 tablespoon of melted butter
- 1/4 cup of quick-cooking oats
- 1 tablespoon of brown sugar
- 1/4 teaspoon of ground cinnamon

Muffins:
- 1 - 1/2 teaspoons of ground cinnamon
- 1 teaspoon of baking powder
- 1 egg, lightly beaten
- 1 teaspoon of vanilla extract
- 1/2 teaspoon of baking soda
- 1/2 teaspoon of salt
- 1 1/2 cups of quick-cooking oats

- 1 1/4 cups of all-purpose flour

- 2 tablespoons of all-purpose flour

- 1/2 cup of brown sugar

- 1/2 cup of unsweetened applesauce

- 1/2 cup of milk

- 1/4 cup of vegetable oil

- 1 apple chopped, peeled and cored

PREPARATIONS

- Preheat oven to 400 degrees F.

- Grease a 12-cup muffin tin and line with paper liners.

- Stir 1 tablespoon of brown sugar, 1/4 cup of oats, 1/4 teaspoon of cinnamon and melted butter together in a small bowl. Set it aside.

- Whisk 1/2 cup of brown sugar, 1 1/2 cups of oats, flour, baking powder, 1 1/2 teaspoons of cinnamon, salt and baking soda together in a large bowl.

- Stir milk, applesauce, oil, egg and vanilla extract together in a bowl.

- Stir applesauce mixture into flour mixture just until all ingredients are moistened.

- Stir in the apple and spoon of apple mixture into prepared muffins cups, for about 2/3 full, sprinkle oat and top mixture evenly over each muffin.

- Bake in the preheated oven, for about 15 minutes until a toothpick inserted near the center comes out clean.

- Serve and enjoy.

NOTE:

Bake the oatmeal cups, cool completely, and store in the refrigerator all week for easy breakfasts. Reheat in the microwave or bake in a 350°F (177°C) oven for 5 - 6 minutes. To freeze, bake and cool oatmeal cups. Cover tightly and freeze for up to 3 months. Thaw in the refrigerator or at room temperature. Warm to your liking.

PREP TIME: 20 mins

COOK TIME: 15 mins

TOTAL TIME: 35 mins

YIELD: 12 muffins

VEGGIE OMELET

Veggie Omelet is one of the easiest and fastest breakfast recipes to eat. It is essential to start your day off right with nutrient-dense vegetables and protein.

This recipe can be prepared and eaten as a side dish or as a full meal. It's so healthy, simply delicious, light and fluffy.

The most interesting part of it is that you can use your favorite vegetables to create your own perfect omelet.

INGREDIENTS

- 4 eggs
- 2 tablespoons of milk
- 3/4 teaspoon of salt
- 2 tablespoons of butter
- 1 small onion, chopped
- 1 green bell pepper, chopped
- 1/8 teaspoon of freshly ground black pepper
- 2 ounces of shredded Swiss cheese

PREPARATIONS

- In a medium skillet, melt 1 tablespoon of butter over medium heat.
- Place bell pepper and onion inside the skillet.
- Cook until vegetables are just tender, for about 5 minutes, stirring occasionally.

- Beat the eggs with 1/2 teaspoon of salt and pepper with milk while the vegetables are cooking.

- In a small bowl, shred the cheese and set it aside.

- Remove the vegetables from the heat.

- Transfer them into a separate bowl and sprinkle the rest of the salt over them.

- Melt the rest of the butter over medium heat.

- Coat the skillet with the butter.

- Add the egg mixture while the butter is bubbly and cook the egg until the eggs begin to set on the bottom of the pan, for about 2 minutes.

- Lift the edges of the omelet gently using a spatula to let the uncooked part of the eggs flows to the edges and cook.

- Continue cooking until the center of the omelet starts to look dry, for about 3 minutes.

- Sprinkle the cheese over the omelet.

- Spoon the vegetable mixture into the center of the omelet.

- Using a spatula gently fold one edge of the omelet, over the vegetables,

- Let the omelet cook until the cheese melts to your desired consistency, for about 2 minutes.

- Slide the omelet out of the skillet and place on a plate.

- Cut into half, serve and enjoy.

NOTE:

Freezer bags are a great option for preserving omelets in either the fridge of the freezer. Store omelets in the fridge for only about 3-4 days. Omelets should be tightly wrapped or sealed in an airtight container or bag. The key to storing them is to make sure they are sealed tightly into whatever storage format you use.

You can preserve omelets by storing it in the freezer for up to 4 months. They will taste the freshest if they are used within 2 months. To store in the freezer, wrap tightly or place into freezer bags or an airtight container. This is just to ensure that they really are sealed tight in the order to preserve the flavor.

PREP TIME: 10 mins

COOK TIME: 15 mins

TOTAL TIME: 25 mins

YIELD: 2 servings

EGG PEPPER CUPS

All you will be needing are eggs, fresh ground pepper, whatever fresh herbs you have on hand and some coloured bell peppers to get your morning meal ready. This is the kind of recipe that is so simple to make-ahead and can be ready to eat within 30 minutes.

Giving this Eggs Pepper Cups a try would be great seriously. An easy breakfast idea that is full of filling protein to take on your day. I call it a morning

energizer.

INGREDIENTS

- 4 large eggs
- Freshly ground pepper and kosher salt
- 4 small multicolored bell peppers
- Chopped fresh herbs

PREPARATIONS

- Preheat oven to 350 degrees F.
- Slice bottom of 2-inches of the pepper (do this for each of the pepper - in 1 piece) to form shallow cups.
- Reserve tops for another use next time.
- Place the pepper on a baking sheet.
- Crack 1 egg into each of the pepper.
- Season with pepper and salt.

- Bake for about 25 minutes, until yolks are still a little runny and whites are firm.

- Sprinkle with chopped fresh herbs of your choice.

- Serve and enjoy.

NOTES:

Keep them all in an airtight container in the refrigerator or place each individual egg muffin cup in a resealable bag for an easy grab-and-go breakfast. Dispose after 6 days. You can also freeze the cooked egg muffins, once cooled, in a resealable bag for up to 3 months.

PREP TIME: 5 mins

COOK TIME: 0 mins

TOTAL TIME: 30 mins

YIELD: 6 pepper cups

VEGGIE FRITTATA

MY **BONUS** RECIPE

Veggie Frittata is just like an open omelet that sure makes a colorful presentation. They are vegetarian meals that are a great way to transform eggs into a more substantial breakfast. You should know that Eggs are naturally rich in protein and low in carbs. So, I believe this is the perfect combo to maintain steady blood-sugar levels.

Start your day with this delicious meal today and enjoy.

INGREDIENTS

- 6 eggs
- 1/4 cup of cilantro chopped
- 1/2 cup of cherry tomatoes sliced
- 1/4 cup of full fat yogurt optional
- 1 cup of mushrooms chopped
- 8-10 stalks asparagus ends trimmed and chopped
- 1 cup of shredded mozzarella cheese divided
- 1/4 cup of red onions chopped

PREPARATIONS

- Preheat the oven to 425 degrees F.
- Whisk together the egg, salt, pepper, half of the shredded mozzarella cheese and yogurt; set mixture aside.
- In a cast iron pan or oven safe pan, heat the olive oil.

- Add mushrooms, onions and asparagus and cook until the vegetables soften for about 5 minutes.

- Pour the egg mixture on top of the cooked vegetables.

- Place sliced cherry tomatoes on top, then add the rest of the cheese.

- Bake in the preheated oven uncovered for about 15 minutes until the center is set and not jiggly.

- Serve and enjoy.

NOTE:

Frittata can be preserved well for a few days in the refrigerator. You can serve leftover frittata chilled, let it come to room temperature on its own, or gently warm individual slices in the microwave or oven.

PREP TIME: 10 mins

COOK TIME: 15 mins

TOTAL TIME: 25 mins

YIELD: 4 servings

COCONUT PORRIDGE

MY **BONUS** RECIPE

According to the medical website WebMD, coconut porridge could help to control blood sugar in diabetes patients. It's better at maintaining blood sugar levels over a longer period of time. It's a food that takes longer to digest and the kind of foods that takes longer to digest are extremely better for diabetes.

Coconut Porridge is one of the most nutritious breakfast dishes you can serve for your entire family in the morning. *Enjoy your morning.*

INGREDIENTS

- 1 ounce of coconut oil or butter
- 4 tablespoons of coconut cream
- 1 beaten egg
- 1 pinch of salt
- 1 tablespoon of coconut flour
- 1 pinch of ground psyllium husk powder

PREPARATIONS

- Combine the coconut flour, egg, psyllium husk powder and salt in a small bowl.
- Melt the butter and coconut cream over low heat.

- Whisk in the egg mixture slowly, combining until you achieve a thick creamy texture.

- Serve with cream or coconut milk.

- Top your porridge with some fresh or frozen berries.

- Serve and enjoy.

NOTE:

Store into lidded containers in the refrigerator for up to 3 days.

PREP TIME: 10 mins

COOK TIME: 0 mins

TOTAL TIME: 10 mins

YIELD: 1 serving

LUNCH RECIPES

TORTILLA CHICKEN SOUP

This recipe delivers the same flavor you love in traditional tortilla soup, but without all high carbs ingredients.

It's so good and perfect for people with diabetics. You can top with crispy tortilla chips and lighten this up by baking the tortilla so you can have heartier recipe. I would suggest you should add lime to give it a zesty freshness. Also, this recipe is for you if you're looking forwards to eating healthy.

INGREDIENTS

- 1 cup of corn, drained if canned
- 2 chicken breasts boneless, skinless
- 1/4 cup of cilantro chopped
- 1 lime juiced
- 1 sliced avocado
- 1 tablespoon of olive oil
- 1 chopped onion
- 3 large cloves garlic, minced
- 1 jalapeño deseeded and diced
- 1 teaspoon of ground cumin
- 1 teaspoon of chili powder
- 14.5 ounces of crushed tomatoes
- 1 can diced tomatoes with chilies

- 3 cups of chicken broth

- 14.5 ounce can black beans, drained and rinsed

Crispy Tortilla Strips

- 1/4 cup of olive oil

- salt

- 6 6-inches corn tortillas cut into 1/4-inch strips

PREPARATIONS

- Over medium high heat, heat 1/4 cup of olive oil in a small pan.

- Add tortilla strips into small batches and then fry till crisp.

- Drain and add sprinkle salt.

- In a large pot over medium heat, heat olive oil and add garlic, onion, jalapeno and onion, then cook until softened.

- Add the rest of the ingredients and simmer until chicken is cooked through, for about 20 minutes.

- Remove chicken and shred it.

- Add it back to the pot and then simmer for just 3 mins.

- Spoon your soup into bowls.

- Top with lime wedges, tortilla strips and sliced avocado.

- Serve and enjoy.

NOTE:

This chicken tortilla soup recipe is perfect for freezing, because it doesn't contain dairy and reheats really well. Cool the soup down completely, then store in a freezer-safe container. It will last in the refrigerator for 3-4 days in an airtight container. To reheat, pour into a saucepan over medium-low heat, stirring until warmed through.

PREP TIME: 10 mins

COOK TIME: 30 mins

TOTAL TIME: 40 mins

YIELD: 8 servings

CHICKEN BROCCOLI SALAD

Chicken Broccoli Salad is just so easy, creamy and simple to make. This healthy meal is the best for you if you're a veggie fan. It is super nutritious and amazingly versatile too. You should ideally keep a safe distance from junk and processed foods if you are a diabetes patient. It is also advisable to avoid sugary foods. This is why I'm introducing this Chicken Broccoli Salad to you.

Enjoy!

INGREDIENTS

- 1/4 cup of apple cider vinegar
- 1/4 cup of white sugar
- 1/4 cup of crumbled cooked bacon
- 8 cups of broccoli florets
- 3 cooked skinless, boneless chicken breast halves, cubed
- 1 cup of chopped walnuts
- 6 green onions, chopped
- 1 cup of mayonnaise

PREPARATIONS

- Combine chicken, broccoli, walnuts and green onions in a large bowl.
- Whisk together vinegar, mayonnaise and sugar in a bowl until it's well blended.

- Pour mayonnaise dressing over broccoli mixture and toss to coat.

- Cover and refrigerate till chilled if you feel like.

- To serve: sprinkle with crumbled bacon.

- Serve and enjoy.

NOTE:

Store, covered, in refrigerator until ready to serve, so that the dressing has time to chill and the flavors blend. The broccoli salad can be kept, covered, in the refrigerator for several days.

PREP TIME: 15 mins

COOK TIME: 0 mins

TOTAL TIME: 1 hour 15 mins

YIELD: 10 servings

BLACK BEAN SALAD

You need to have a taste of different salad every day. This Black Bean Salad is a very tasty and satisfying lunch salad. I love this combination of veggies and beans. It's a complete meal that is tasty, healthy and super easy to make.

The most interesting part of this meal is its excellent when cold or heated. *So good!*

INGREDIENTS

- 1 avocado, deseeded, peeled and cut into chunks
- 1/2 to 1 teaspoon of sugar (to taste)
- Salt and pepper to taste
- 1/2 cup of chopped fresh cilantro
- 1 1/2 cups of freshly cooked black beans (or 1 (15 ounces) can of black beans, drained and rinsed)
- 1 1/2 cups of frozen corn, defrosted (or fresh corn, drained, parboiled and cooled, or cooled and grilled)
- 1/2 cup of shallots or chopped green onions (including onion greens)
- 2 tablespoons of lime juice (about the juice from one lime)
- 1 tablespoon of extra virgin olive oil
- 1/2 fresh jalapeño pepper, minced and deseeded, or 1/2 pickled jalapeño pepper, minced (not seeded)
- 3 fresh plum tomatoes, deseeded and chopped and/or 1 red bell pepper, chopped and deseeded

PREPARATIONS

- Combine the corn, black beans, minced jalapenos, chopped green onions, chopped tomatoes or red bell pepper, olive oil and lime juice in a large bowl.

- Fold in the chopped avocado gently.

- Add pepper and salt to taste.

- Sprinkle with sugar to taste (sugar that is enough to balance the acidity from the lime juice).

- Chill before serving.

- Add the chopped fresh cilantro.

- Serve and enjoy.

NOTE:

To preserve, refrigerate the bean salad in airtight containers. Properly stored, bean salad will last for 3 to 5 days in the refrigerator.

PREP TIME: 20 mins

COOK TIME: 0 mins

TOTAL TIME: 20 mins

YIELD: 6 servings

KALE SALAD WITH LEMON DRESSING

This is a vegetarian, low-carb salad that might not sound like a filling meal, but this is loaded with leafy greens and protein that will power you through your day. As we all know, kale is one of those foods that is incredibly healthy, but most people are always afraid to try. Taking a step to try this recipe is a great way to get more vegetables into your diet. This Kale Salad with Lemon Dressing is delicious and actually easy to prepare.

INGREDIENTS

Lemon Dressing

- 1 minced garlic clove
- 1 teaspoon of dried oregano
- 1/2 cup of extra virgin olive oil
- 1/4 cup of lemon juice
- Salt and pepper to taste

Kale Salad

- 1/2 red onion thinly sliced
- 1/2 cup of crumbled feta cheese
- 1-pint cherry or grape tomatoes halved
- 1 large bunch of about 10 ounces (or 3-4 cups of kale leaves), finely chopped
- 1 cucumber deseeded and diced

PREPARATIONS

Making the Lemon Dressing:

- Combine together the lemon juice, garlic, olive oil, salt, oregano and pepper in a small or medium mixing bowl.

- Whisk until well combined.

Making the Kale Salad:

- Add together all the chopped ingredients in a large bowl and combine.

- Pour the dressing over the salad and mix together.

- Sprinkle with some feta cheese just before serving.

- You can store your dressed and prepared salad in the fridge for up to 2 days.

- Serve and enjoy.

NOTE:

You can store this salad in an airtight container in the fridge for up to 7 days.

PREP TIME: 10 mins

COOK TIME: 0 mins

TOTAL TIME: 10 mins

YIELD: 4 servings

CARROT GINGER SOUP

Carrot Ginger Soup is an easy make-ahead meal and a great way to add some fiber-packed and nutritious vegetables to your diet. If you have diabetes, the more vegetables you eat, the better. This meal is low in carbs and calories, which is a must have for people with diabetes.

It's full of lots of the good stuff your body needs, such as vitamins, antioxidants, minerals and even fiber. This meal does not only offer fragrance and color but it's light and soothing as well.

INGREDIENTS

- 1 tablespoon of apple cider vinegar
- 3 to 4 cups of vegetable broth
- Sea salt and fresh black pepper
- 1 tablespoon of extra-virgin olive oil
- 1 cup of chopped yellow onions
- 3 garlic cloves, smashed
- 2 heaping cups of chopped carrots
- 1 - 1/2 teaspoons of grated fresh ginger
- 1 teaspoon of maple syrup, or to taste (optional)
- coconut milk for garnish, optional
- dollops of pesto, optional

PREPARATIONS

- In a large pot, heat the olive oil over medium heat.

- Add the onions and a pinch of salt and pepper.

- Cook until softened, stirring occasionally, for about 8 minutes.

- Add the smashed garlic cloves and the chopped carrots into the pot.

- Cook for another 8 minutes, stirring occasionally.

- Stir in the ginger and add the apple cider vinegar.

- The next thing you'll want to do is add 3 to 4 cups of broth.

- Reduce to a simmer and cook for about 30 minutes, until the carrots are soft.

- Let it cool slightly and transfer into a blender.

- Blend until smooth.

- Taste and adjust seasonings.

- Add maple syrup if you feel like.

- Serve with a dollop of pesto or drizzle of coconut milk.

- Enjoy.

NOTE:

Leftover carrot ginger soup can be frozen for a quick and simple meal later. Although creamed soups sometimes separate when you defrost and reheat them due to the cream base, it can be remedied with careful blending. If you're freezing the soup, let it cool to room temperature and then transfer it too quart-sized freezer bags (the sturdy ones please). Freeze these flat and then they stack nicely in your fridge. Reheating the soup is easy. Let it thaw slowly or dunk it in warm water for a faster thaw.

PREP TIME: 15 mins

COOK TIME: 30 mins

TOTAL TIME: 45 mins

YIELD: 4 servings

SHRIMP SALAD

Shrimp salad is a perfect light lunch. Loaded with healthy ingredients like black pepper, onion, celery and kosher salt. I'm sure it combines all of your favorite ingredients in one bowl, right?

This is a satisfying dish that has all of the crunch with much less fat. When you have a bite, you bite into a perfectly crispy shrimp salad.

INGREDIENTS

For the Salad:

- Freshly ground black pepper
- 1/4 finely chopped red onion
- 1 finely chopped stalk celery
- 1 pound of shrimp, deveined and peeled
- 1 tablespoon of extra-virgin olive oil
- Kosher salt
- 2 tablespoons of freshly chopped dill
- Toasted bread or butterhead or romaine lettuce, for serving

For the Dressing:

- 1/2 cup of mayonnaise
- Juice and zest of 1 lemon
- 1 teaspoon of Dijon mustard

PREPARATIONS

- Preheat oven to 400 degrees F.

- Toss shrimp with oil on a large baking sheet.

- Season with pepper and salt.

- Bake for about 5 minutes, until shrimp are completely opaque.

- Whisk together mayonnaise, zest, lemon juice and Dijon in a large bowl.

- Season with pepper and salt.

- Add your cooked shrimp, celery, red onion and dill to bowl.

- Then toss until well combined.

- Serve over lettuce and enjoy.

NOTE:

This will last up to 3 days in the fridge when preserved properly in an airtight container.

PREP TIME: 5 mins

COOK TIME: 0 mins

TOTAL TIME: 20 mins

YIELD: 2 servings

CRISPY TOFU

MY **BONUS** RECIPE

This is one of the best crispy tofu recipes for lunch. It uses little oil and it's baked to perfection. It can be perfect for just snacking on!

It's really easy to make, so crispy and it's made with healthy ingredients. The sesame oil used in this recipe gives it a very nice flavor (by the way, you can use avocado / olive oil - it's your choice).

I hope you'll enjoy it.

INGREDIENTS

- 1/4 teaspoon of garlic powder
- 1/4 teaspoon of pure maple syrup
- 1/4 teaspoon of rice wine vinegar
- 1 tablespoon of toasted sesame oil, or your favorite oil
- 1 (14 ounces) container extra firm tofu, pressed and patted dry for at least 15 minutes
- 1 teaspoon of soy sauce or tamari
- 2 teaspoons of corn starch or arrowroot powder

PREPARATIONS

- Preheat oven to 400 degrees F.
- Whisk together tamari or soy sauce, sesame oil, maple syrup, garlic powder and vinegar in a medium sized bowl.
- Cut the press tofu into bite sized pieces.

- Place the pieces into the oil mixture.

- Stir the tofu using a spoon or spatula, making sure it's completely coated.

- Sprinkle 1 teaspoon of the arrowroot powder over it and mix well till all of the tofu is coated.

- Sprinkle the rest of the arrowroot powder and mix carefully just until you can't see the dry white powder anymore.

- Using parchment paper or nonstick to line a large baking sheet.

- Pour the tofu onto baking sheet and arrange it so that the pieces won't be touching each other.

- Bake tofu until crispy and golden, for about 25 minutes, stirring 2 to 3 times during the baking.

- Let the tofu sit for some minutes to crisp even more before enjoying.

- Serve and enjoy.

NOTE:

While crispy tofu is slightly seasoned, it does still benefit from a sauce. Best when fresh but can be stored in the refrigerator for up to 3 days. Reheat in a 375 degrees F (190 C) oven until very hot.

PREP TIME: 15 mins

COOK TIME: 30 mins

TOTAL TIME: 35 mins

YIELD: 4 servings

SPINACH SOUP WITH PESTO & CHICKEN

MY **BONUS** RECIPE

This soup is from Italy. It's a fragrant flavored soup that takes advantage of quick cooking ingredients. It features a simple homemade pesto which adds a fresh herb flavor to the meal.

You can substitute about 3 tablespoons of store-bought pesto if you can't wait to prepare this meal. Prepare, serve and enjoy!

INGREDIENTS

- 1 large clove garlic, minced
- 1/8 cup of lightly packed fresh basil leaves
- Freshly ground pepper to taste
- 5 cups of reduced-sodium chicken broth
- 1 1/2 teaspoons of dried marjoram
- 6 ounces of baby spinach, coarsely chopped
- 2 teaspoons with 1 tablespoon of extra-virgin olive oil, divided
- 1/2 cup of carrot or diced red bell pepper
- 1 large boneless, skinless chicken breast (about 8 ounces), cut into quarters
- 1 15-ounces can of cannellini beans or great northern beans, rinsed
- 1/4 cup of grated Parmesan cheese

- 3/4 cup of plain or herbed multigrain croutons for garnish (optional)

PREPARATIONS

- In a large saucepan, heat 2 tablespoons of oil over medium high heat.

- Add carrot or bell pepper with chicken together.

- Cook, turning the chicken and stirring occasionally, for about 3 minutes, until the chicken begins to brown.

- Add garlic and cook, stirring, for another 1 minute.

- Stir in marjoram and broth.

- Bring to a boil over high heat and reduce the heat.

- Simmer, stirring occasionally, for about 5 minutes until the chicken is cooked through.

- Transfer the chicken pieces to a clean cutting board to cool using a slotted spoon.

- Add beans and spinach into the pot, then bring to a boil.

- Cook for 5 mins to blend the flavors.

- In a food processor, combine the parmesan, 1 tablespoon of oil, basil.

- Process until a coarse paste forms, adding a little water and scrape down the sides.

- Cut the chicken into small size pieces.

- Stir the pesto and chicken into the pot.

- Season with pepper and heat until it's hot.

- Garnish with croutons, if you feel like.

- Serve and enjoy.

NOTE:

Store in a clean container wrapped with paper towels for 3 to 5 days. Place it in the refrigerator in the crisp drawer to save the greens for up to ten days. Paper towels absorb the moisture and keep it fresh.

PREP TIME: 10 mins

COOK TIME: 20 mins

TOTAL TIME: 30 mins

YIELD: 5 servings

DINNER RECIPES

FRENCH LENTILS

This is one of my favorite Diabetic Dinner Recipes because it helps stabilize your blood sugar levels. French Lentils are full of complex carbs that can help you with 25% of protein if you have diabetes.

French Lentils also improves the flow of blood, prevents heart disease and protects the artery walls.

INGREDIENTS

- 2 1/4 cups of French lentils
- 3 tablespoons of olive or vegetable oil
- 1 teaspoon of dried or fresh thyme
- 3 bay leaves
- 1 tablespoon of kosher salt
- 1 onion, peeled and finely chopped
- 2 cloves garlic, peeled and finely chopped
- 1 carrot, peeled and finely chopped

PREPARATIONS

- Place a large saucepan over a medium heat and add oil.
- Add chopped vegetables when hot and sauté for about 5 to 10 minutes, until softened.
- Add lentils, 6 cups of water, thyme, salt and bay leaves.
- Bring to a boil and reduce to a fast simmer.
- Simmer for 20 to 25 minutes until they are tender and have absorbed most of the water.

61

- Drain any excess water after lentils have cooked, if necessary.

- Serve immediately and enjoy.

NOTE:

Properly stored, cooked lentils will last for 3 to 5 days in the refrigerator. Cooked lentils should be discarded if left out for more than 2 hours at room temperature.

PREP TIME: 15 mins

COOK TIME: 25 mins

TOTAL TIME: 40 mins

YIELD: 4 servings

CHICKEN FAJITAS

This is a delicious Chicken Fajitas recipe that is super great for a weeknight meal. They are loaded with lots of light ingredients, flavor and are perfect if you're following diabetes diet.

They are easy and quick to make, and cleanup is pretty fast too.

INGREDIENTS

- 2 teaspoons of fajita seasoning
- 1 green bell pepper, cut into strips
- 1 red bell pepper, cut into strips
- 1 clove garlic, minced
- 1 cup of sliced onion
- 2 boneless, skinless chicken breasts, cut into strips
- 4 low-carb whole wheat tortillas, warmed

PREPARATIONS

- Cooking spray to coat a large skillet.
- Cook garlic, bell peppers and onion over medium heat until tender, for about 6 to 8 minutes, stirring occasionally.
- Remove to a plate.
- Add chicken and fajita seasoning; cook until no longer pink in center, for about 5 minutes.
- Return vegetables to skillet and cook until heated through, for about 2 to 4 more minutes.

- Divide fajita mixture evenly onto tortillas.

- Serve immediately and enjoy.

NOTE:

When stored in the refrigerator in an air-tight container, this recipe can easily last up to 4-6 days, which makes chicken a great choice for your meal prep.

PREP TIME: 10 mins

COOK TIME: 15 mins

TOTAL TIME: 25 mins

YIELD: 4 servings

VEGGIE RICE

Rice is high in carbohydrates, but some types of rice like brown rice, are a whole grain food.

This kind of Veggie Rice is extremely high in carbs because it's loaded with veggies. Adding vegetables not only enhances its vitamin value but also contributes lots of fiber that prevents a quick rise in blood sugar levels after a meal.

INGREDIENTS

- 4 tablespoons of oil
- 2 cups of water
- 1 cup of basmati rice
- 1 small onion finely chopped
- 1/2 cup of frozen veggies. You can use a mix of corn, carrots, peas and green beans
- Salt and pepper to taste.

PREPARATIONS

- Heat the oil in a pot and fry the onion till translucent.
- Add the pepper, frozen veggies, salt and cook for 5 minutes.
- Add the water, and use lid to cover the pot.
- Bring water to a boil and then add the rice.
- Cook on medium high heat till rice is almost cooked and most of the water has evaporated.
- Lower the heat and cover the rice.

- Let the rice steam until it's completely cooked, for about 5 minutes.

- Remove from heat and use fork to fluff the rice.

- Serve immediately.

- Enjoy.

NOTE:

To preserve veggie rice, it is best to freeze it as soon as possible after cooking. Pack the veggie rice into a microwavable container as soon as it is cooked. When cooled, seal the container and place into the freezer. You can keep rice in the freezer for up to one month and it will still retain its moisture and taste, but you shouldn't leave it in the freezer much longer than that.

PREP TIME: 5 mins

COOK TIME: 20 mins

TOTAL TIME: 25 mins

YIELD: 4 servings

GRILLED TUNA KEBABS

Try Grilled Tuna Kebabs when you're looking to cook out. It's packed with fresh herbs and lime juice that brighten these skewers of tuna.

Enjoy the warm weather with this healthy grilled tuna kebabs recipe. They are a smart choice if you follow a diabetic diet, and so delicious enough for the whole family.

INGREDIENTS

- 3 tablespoons of fresh lime juice (from 2 limes)
- freshly ground pepper and coarse salt.
- 1 1/2 pounds of sushi-grade yellowfin tuna (cut into 1 1/2-inch cubes)
- 1/4 cup plus 2 tablespoons of extra-virgin olive oil
- 3 tablespoons of chopped fresh cilantro

PREPARATIONS

- Heat a grill pan over medium heat.
- Toss tuna with 1 tablespoon of oil.
- Thread tuna onto 4 kebabs.
- Combine lime juice, cilantro and 1/4 cup of oil.
- Season with pepper and salt.
- Reserve about 3 tablespoons.
- Brush pan with the remaining tablespoon of oil.

- Grill tuna, turning kebabs and brushing tuna occasionally with lime sauce, for about 2 minutes per side for rare or to desired doneness.

- Transfer kebabs to a serving plate.

- Brush with reserved lime sauce.

- Serve immediately and enjoy.

NOTE:

If it has been sitting out for more than two hours at room temperature, toss it. On a hotter day (above 90 degrees Fahrenheit), make that one hour. If you haven't exceeded the time limit, then place it in a shallow pan being careful not to over pack it. Cover and place near the top of the refrigerator. Eat within a few days or toss.

PREP TIME: 15 mins

COOK TIME: 0 mins

TOTAL TIME: 20 mins

YIELD: 4 servings

SPICY TURKEY TACOS

Tacos can be tasty and permissible in your diet. Add as many veggies you can to top it. It is a very versatile recipe that uses ground turkey to lower calories. It also makes for light and healthy tacos, simple and plain.

This Tacos recipe is also easy to prepare, healthy and delicious at the same time. Are you looking for Dinner recipe that is full of flavor? then this is the right recipe for you. Try it and you would be wowed!

INGREDIENTS

- 1/2 teaspoon of ground cumin
- 2 cups of shredded lettuce
- 8 taco shells
- 1/2 teaspoon of dried oregano
- 1/2 teaspoon of paprika
- 1/2 teaspoon of ground cinnamon
- 1 pound of extra-lean ground turkey
- 1 small red onion, finely chopped
- 1 cup of salsa
- 1/2 cup of shredded pepper jack cheese
- 1/4 cup of fat-free sour cream
- Cubed avocado and extra salsa, optional

PREPARATIONS

- Heat taco shells just according to the directions in the package.

- Cook turkey and onion in a large nonstick skillet over medium heat until the meat is no longer pink.

- Stir in spices and salsa.

- Heat through and serve immediately.

- Fill each of the taco shell with 1/3 cup of turkey mixture if you want to serve.

- Serve with cheese, lettuce or sour cream if you feel like.

- Enjoy.

NOTE:

To preserve this lovely recipe, cool completely and then measure into Ziploc freezer bags. Be sure to remove all of the air from the bag before sealing. Label the bag and the amount of Taco Meat you put into the bag. To thaw it, just pull it out of the freezer and let it thaw overnight in the fridge. Or you can run the bag under cold water until it is loosened up enough to dump out of the bag. Heat on the stovetop or in the microwave and use.

PREP TIME: 15 mins

COOK TIME: 0 mins

TOTAL TIME: 25 mins

YIELD: 4 servings

LIME QUINOA WITH CILANTRO

Quinoa has more protein than any other grain. This is a refreshing recipe that tastes good and makes up for a filling dinner as well. Apart from being very nutritious, quinoa has a very low glycemic index and gluten free which helps in keeping blood sugar under control.

The good news about this recipe is it even helps in reducing weight and it's full of refreshing flavor.

INGREDIENTS

- 1 mango, diced and peeled
- 1 diced jalapeno pepper
- 1/4 teaspoon of salt
- 1 avocado - peeled, pitted, and diced
- 1 1/2 tablespoons of lime juice
- 2 tablespoons of chopped fresh cilantro
- 1 tablespoon of olive oil
- 2 cloves garlic, minced
- 1/2 red onion, diced
- 1 cup of quinoa, rinsed and drained
- 1 1/2 cups of low-sodium chicken broth
- 1 cup of corn

PREPARATIONS

- In a saucepan, heat olive oil over medium heat

- Cook and stir garlic until fragrant for about 1 minute.

- Add jalapeno pepper, onion and salt.

- Cook and stir for about 5 to 10 minutes, until onion is tender.

- Add quinoa and cook for 2 minutes until slightly browned.

- Pour in the chicken broth, then bring to a boil.

- Reduce heat to low and simmer for about 15 minutes until broth is absorbed.

- Stir mango, corn, lime juice, avocado and cilantro into the quinoa mixture.

- Serve immediately and enjoy.

NOTE:

Consider freezing the leftovers for an easy side for future meals. Just let the quinoa cool completely before freezing.

PREP TIME: 20 mins

COOK TIME: 25 mins

TOTAL TIME: 45 mins

YIELD: 6 servings

POTATOES WITH ROASTED VEGGIES

MY **BONUS** RECIPE

Do you know you can have a healthy serving of roasted veggies with potatoes? This recipe is loaded with veggies that is so easy to prepare. It can be made a day ahead. What you have to do the next day is just 'reheat' before serving. You can use lemon juice if you don't have balsamic vinegar on hand. By the way, people with diabetes should be mindful of the portions of potato they consume. It shouldn't be too much.

INGREDIENTS

- 1 red onion, quartered
- 1 tablespoon of chopped fresh thyme
- 2 tablespoons of chopped fresh rosemary
- 1/4 cup of olive oil
- 2 tablespoons of balsamic vinegar
- 1 small butternut squash, cubed
- 2 red bell peppers, deseeded and diced
- 1 sweet potato, peeled and cubed
- 3 Yukon Gold potatoes, cubed
- salt and freshly ground black pepper

PREPARATIONS

- Preheat oven to 475 degrees F.

- Combine the red bell peppers, squash, Yukon gold potatoes and sweet potato in a large bowl.

- Separate the red onion quarters into pieces, then add them into the mixture.

- Stir together rosemary, thyme, vinegar, salt, olive oil, pepper and salt in a small bowl.

- Toss with vegetables till they're coated.

- Spread evenly on a large roasting pan.

- Roast for about 35 minutes in the preheated oven, until vegetables are cooked through and browned, turn the vegetables every 10 minutes.

- Serve and enjoy.

NOTE:

Refrigerate the potatoes in shallow airtight containers or resealable plastic bags. Properly stored, cooked potatoes with roasted veggies will last for 3 to 5 days in the refrigerator.

PREP TIME: 15 mins

COOK TIME: 40 mins

TOTAL TIME: 55 mins

YIELD: 12 servings

MUSHROOM STROGANOFF

MY **BONUS** RECIPE

The picture may not look appetizing but it's just so good. This is a diabetic recipe that is so rich, thick and can be eaten for dinner.

This recipe makes a great meal for diabetics as they contain very low amount of carbs, which means they don't raise blood sugar levels. They also have a very low glycaemic index.

INGREDIENTS

- 3 cloves garlic, minced
- 4 teaspoons of chopped fresh thyme
- 2 1/2 tablespoons of all-purpose flour
- 2 cups of beef stock
- 2 tablespoons of chopped fresh parsley leaves
- 8 ounces of medium pasta shells
- 3 tablespoons of unsalted butter
- 1 1/2 pounds of cremini mushrooms, thinly sliced
- 2 large shallots, diced
- Kosher salt and freshly ground black pepper, to taste
- 1 1/2 teaspoons of Dijon mustard
- 3/4 cup of sour cream
- 2/3 cup of freshly grated Parmesan

PREPARATIONS

- Cook pasta according to package instructions in a large pot of boiling salted water. Drain it well.

- In a large skillet, melt butter over medium high heat.

- Add shallots and mushrooms and cook, stirring occasionally, until mushrooms are browned and tender, for about 5 minutes.

- Season with pepper and salt, to taste.

- Stir in thyme and garlic, cook for 1 minute, until fragrant.

- Whisk in flour cook for 1 minute, until lightly browned.

- Whisk in beef stock and Dijon gradually and bring it to a boil.

- Reduce heat and simmer, stirring occasionally, until slightly thickened and reduced, for about 5 minutes.

- Stir in sour cream and pasta until heated through, for about 2 minutes.

- Stir in Parmesan for 1 minute, until melted.

- Stir in parsley, season with pepper and salt, to taste.

- Serve immediately and enjoy.

NOTE:

This vegan mushroom stroganoff sauce keeps in the refrigerator for 2 to 3 days or can be frozen for up to 2 months. I recommend storing or freeze the sauce separately from the pasta in a sealed container. When ready to serve, defrost overnight in the fridge, then heat it up on the stovetop and serve with your favorite side and fresh herbs.

PREP TIME: 10 mins

COOK TIME: 20 mins

TOTAL TIME: 30 mins

YIELD : 4 servings

DESSERT RECIPES

SUGAR FREE BUCKEYE BALLS

These delicious tasting Sugar Free Buckeye Balls are the perfect treat to share with your families and friends. They are low in carbs and diabetic friendly, because it's made with zero sugar.

We'll be adding a Sugar Free Peanut butter to this recipe. They actually work together in creating delicious taste.

INGREDIENTS

- 6 cups of Sugar Free Powdered Sugar
- 1 teaspoon of Vanilla Extract
- 1 1/2 cups of Sugar Free Peanut Butter
- 1 cup of Butter very soft
- 4 cups of Sugar Free Chocolate Chips

PREPARATIONS

- Prepare a baking sheet with wax paper. Set it aside.
- Cream together the sugar-free peanut butter, vanilla extract and sugar free powdered sugar in a mixing bowl.
- Form the mixture into 1 - 1 1/2-inches balls by rolling the dough in your hands.
- Place each of the ball on the wax prepared baking sheet.
- Place the prepared balls into the freezer for about 25 minutes, until hard.
- Melt the chocolate in a microwave when you're ready to dip the balls in the chocolate or using the double boiler method.

- Stir well as the chocolate melts.

- Remove the peanut butter balls from the freezer and dip each of it into the chocolate. You can leave the area around where you put your toothpick.

- Then place each ball back onto the wax paper and refrigerate them.

- Melt more if you run low on chocolate.

- Serve and enjoy.

NOTE:

The buckeye balls should be stored in an airtight container in the refrigerator to keep them nice and fresh. Stored in this way, they will keep for about 1 month. You can also freeze buckeyes in an airtight container or freezer Ziploc bag for up to 3 months.

PREP TIME: 20 mins

FREEZING TIME: 35 mins

TOTAL TIME: 55 mins

YIELD : 36 balls

PEANUT BUTTER COOKIES

I believe a healthy diet should absolutely include dessert. So if you're looking for the best cookie to enjoy, this Peanut Butter cookies are a healthy way to satisfy your cookie craving after having your breakfast or lunch meal.

They taste good and they come together in a bowl with just 2 ingredients for a super treat.

INGREDIENTS

- 1/2 teaspoon of baking soda
- 1/2 teaspoon of vanilla essence
- 1 cup of smooth peanut butter (no added sugar)
- 1 large egg
- 2/3 cup of erythritol

PREPARATIONS

- Preheat oven to 350 degrees F.
- Line a cookie tray with baking paper and set it aside.
- Add the erythritol to a blender and blend until powdered. Set it aside. (Skip this step if using a confectioner's low carb sweetener).
- In a medium mixing bowl, add all of the ingredients and mix until smooth and glossy dough forms.
- Roll about 2 tablespoons of dough in your palms to form a ball, and place on the prepared cookie tray. Repeat until you consume the doughs. You will end up with 12 to 14 cookies.
- Use a fork to flatten the cookies and create a criss cross patten across the top.

- Bake the cookies for about 12 minutes.

- Remove from the oven and allow it to cool on the baking tray, for about 25 minutes.

- Transfer into a cooling rack for another 15 minutes.

- Serve and enjoy.

NOTE:

At room temperature, you can store these cookies in an airtight container for up to 4 to 6 days (they will last past that point, they just won't be as good). In the freezer, these cookies can be frozen in an airtight container or freezer bag up to 3 months.

PREP TIME: 5 mins

COOK TIME: 15 mins

COOLING TIME: 40 mins

TOTAL TIME: 1 hour

YIELD: 12 balls

CHOCOLATE FUDGE

MY **BONUS** RECIPE

Chocolate Fudge is a simple recipe you can make. It's vegan, low carb, keto and even diabetic friendly.

It can be ready to eat with just 3 to 5 simple ingredients. You just have to let it set very well in the fridge for some hours. I hope you enjoy it!

INGREDIENTS

- 10 ounces of bittersweet chocolate chips
- *Optional:* coarse or flaked sea salt for topping
- 1 1/2 cups of coconut butter
- 1 (13.66 FL ounces) can of full-fat coconut milk

PREPARATIONS

- Use paper or foil to line an 8 by 8 inch baking pan.
- Melt the coconut butter in a small saucepan over low heat.
- Stir in the chocolate chips and coconut milk.
- Cook over low heat, stirring consistently, until the chocolate chips are melted.
- Pour the mixture into the pan.
- Place in refrigerator for about 2 hours, until set.
- Slice, serve and enjoy.

NOTE:

Place the wrapped chocolate fudge inside an airtight container for additional protection from moisture loss, which may cause fudge to become dry and crumbly. Store at room temperature for two to three weeks. Transfer it to the refrigerator if you plan to store it for longer.

PREP TIME: 5 mins

COOK TIME: 2 hours

TOTAL TIME: 2 hours 5 mins

YIELD: 40 squares

LOW-CARB CHEESECAKE

MY **BONUS** RECIPE

This is a healthy low carb cheesecake that is simply delicious and so simple to make. This recipe would definitely satisfy your cheesecake cravings.

This dessert is so healthy that you can eat it as a snack whenever you feel like without feeling guilty at all. It's just so perfect. A perfect recipe for a mid-morning snack or after your workout (before morning meal.)

INGREDIENTS

- 1 tablespoon of Stevia
- 1 teaspoon of vanilla extract
- 8.5 ounces of low fat cottage cheese
- 2 egg whites
- 1 scoop of vanilla protein powder
- 1 serving sugar-free Strawberry Jell-O
- Water

PREPARATIONS

- Preheat the oven to 325 degrees F.
- Prepare the Jell-O according to the instructions on the package.
- Place in the freezer.

- Blend egg whites and cottage cheese until the consistency is smooth.

- Pour the blended mixture inside the bowl.

- Whisk it together with the stevia, protein powder and vanilla extract.

- Transfer the batter into a small nonstick pan, then bake for about 25 minutes.

- Turn off the oven (but let the cake in it cool down).

- Remove the cheesecake once the oven has cooled.

- Pour it over the cheesecake when the Jell-O is almost set.

- Let the cake set in the fridge for about 10 hours before enjoying.

- Now you can serve and enjoy.

NOTE:

Simply slice the pieces of cheesecake and place them on individual pieces of plastic wrap. Wrap them tight, place in a freezer bag or bowl, and store them in the freezer for up to 2 weeks. Any longer than 2 weeks and they will lose quality.

PREP TIME: 10 mins

COOK TIME: 50 mins

TOTAL TIME: 1 hour

YIELD: 2 servings

30 DAYS DIABETIC MEAL PLAN
FOR BEGINNERS

DIABETIC MEAL PLAN (DAYS 1 - 7)

DAY	BREAKFAST	LUNCH	DINNER
1	Mini Veggie Quiche	Chicken Tortilla Soup	French Lentils
2	Shakshuka	Leftover Chicken Tortilla Soup	Leftover French Lentils
3	Leftover Shakshuka	Chicken Broccoli Salad	Veggie Rice
4	Healthy Granola	Black Bean Salad	Chicken Fajitas
5	Leftover Healthy Granola	Leftover Chicken Tortilla Soup	Leftover Veggie Rice
6	Cinnamon Oat Muffins with Apple	Leftover Black Bean Salad	Leftover Chicken Fajitas
7	Leftover Healthy Granola	Chicken Broccoli Salad	Leftover French Lentils

DIABETIC MEAL PLAN (DAYS 8 - 14)

DAY	BREAKFAST	LUNCH	DINNER
8	Veggie Frittata	Kale Salad with Lemon Dressing	Grilled Tuna Kebabs
9	Veggie Omelet	Carrot Ginger Soup	Spicy Turkey Tacos
10	Leftover Veggie Frittata	Leftover Kale Salad with Lemon Dressing	Leftover Grilled Tuna Kebabs
11	Egg Pepper Cups	Shrimp Salad	Lime Quinoa with Cilantro
12	Leftover Egg Pepper Cups	Leftover Carrot Ginger Soup	Leftover Lime Quinoa with Cilantro
13	Leftover Egg Pepper Cups	Leftover Kale Salad with Lemon Dressing	Mushroom Stroganoff
14	Leftover Veggie Omelet	Leftover Shrimp Salad	Leftover Mushroom Stroganoff

DIABETIC MEAL PLAN (DAYS 15 - 21)

DAY	BREAKFAST	LUNCH	DINNER
15	Cinnamon Oat Muffins With Apple	Crispy Tofu	Potatoes with Roasted Veggies
16	Leftover Cinnamon Oat Muffins With Apple	Spinach Soup with Pesto & Chicken	Leftover Potatoes with Roasted Veggies
17	Coconut Porridge	Leftover Crispy Tofu	French Lentils
18	Mini Veggie Quiche	Tortilla Chicken Soup	Veggie Rice
19	Leftover Coconut Porridge	Chicken Broccoli Salad	Leftover French Lentils
20	Leftover Cinnamon Oat Muffins With Apple	Black Bean Salad	Leftover Veggie Rice
21	Leftover Coconut Porridge	Kale Salad With Lemon Dressing	Leftover Veggie Rice

DIABETIC MEAL PLAN (DAYS 22 - 30)

DAY	BREAKFAST	LUNCH	DINNER
22	Healthy Granola	Tortilla Chicken Soup	Potatoes with Roasted Veggies
23	Veggie Omelet	Leftover Tortilla Chicken Soup	French Lentils
24	Shakshuka	Kale Salad With Lemon Dressing	Leftover Potatoes with Roasted Veggies
25	Mini Veggie Quiche	Black Bean Salad	Chicken Fajitas
26	Leftover Veggie Omelet	Carrot Ginger Soup	Leftover French Lentils
27	Leftover Mini Veggie Quiche	Shrimp Salad	Veggie Rice
28	Leftover Shakshuka	Leftover Carrot Ginger Soup	Grilled Tuna Kebabs
29	Veggie Frittata	Leftover Shrimp Salad	Leftover Veggie Rice
30	Leftover Veggie Frittata	Crispy Tofu	Leftover Grilled Tuna Kebabs

THANK YOU!
DIABETIC MEAL PREP
FOR BEGINNERS

CPSIA information can be obtained
at www.ICGtesting.com
Printed in the USA
BVHW070810111120
593051BV00017B/1089